Gymnema

Natural Ayurvedic Herb for Diabetes

Maren Barney

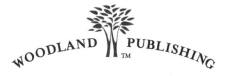

Copyright © 2006 by Woodland Publishing

All rights reserved. No part of this publication may be reproduced, stored in a retrieval system, or transmitted in any form without the prior written permission of the copyright owner.

For permissions, ordering information, or bulk quantity discounts, please contact: Woodland Publishing, 448 East 800 North, Orem, Utah 84097
Visit our Web site: www.woodlandpublishing.com
Toll-free number: (800) 777-2665

The information in this book is for educational purposes only and is not recommended as a means of diagnosing or treating an illness. All matters concerning physical and mental health should be supervised by a health practitioner knowledgeable in treating that particular condition. Neither the publisher nor the author directly or indirectly dispenses medical advice, nor do they prescribe any remedies or assume any responsibility for those who choose to treat themselves.

Cataloging-in-publication data is available from the Library of Congress.

ISBN-13: 978-1-58054-462-7
ISBN-10: 1-58054-462-2

Printed in the United States of America

06   07   08   09   10   1   2   3   4   5   6   7   8   9   10

Contents

Introduction to Ayurveda 5

History of Ayurveda   6

Gymnema (*Gymnema sylvestre*) 11

What Is Diabetes? 12

Symptoms of Diabetes 13

Diagnosing Diabetes 13

Risk Factors for Diabetes 14

Types of Diabetes 14

Managing Blood Glucose Levels 16

Treating Diabetes 18

Long-Term Complications 18

Caring for Yourself 19

Gymnema and Other Conditions 20

Gymnema Dosage 20

Precautions 20

Herbs Commonly Used to Control Blood Sugar Levels 21

Other Herbs Used to Control Blood Sugar Levels 23

References 27

Introduction to Ayurveda

Ayurvedic medicine is a system of health care practiced in India and Sri Lanka that dates back almost four thousand years. It is an approach to wellness and prevention where each person is treated as an individual. The ayurvedic practitioner treats the person, not just the condition or disease.

In ayurvedic tradition, health is a whole-person concept consisting of spiritual as well as physical influences. The focus is not only to cure diseases, but to prevent them and create health and well-being.

This approach differs from that of Western medicine, which tends to regard human bodies as all essentially the same and attempts to treat the condition and its symptoms as opposed to the patient as an individual.

Western medicine tends to view all bodies as having the same physiological makeup and prescribes patients suffering from similar conditions (e.g., cancer) similar treatments (e.g., chemotherapy) regardless of a person's mental or spiritual condition.

The ayurvedic approach recognizes that all illnesses affect the body *and* the mind. Although Western medicine

6 • Gymnema

includes psychologists and psychiatrists, they are generally kept separate from the doctors who treat physical ailments. Ayurvedic practitioners believe that what affects the body affects the mind, and vice versa. According to this philosophy, physical and psychological ailments cannot be separated.

History of Ayurveda

Ayurveda is a Sanskrit word derived from two roots: *ayus* for "life," and *vid*, for "knowledge," translating to "wisdom of life."

Ayus represents a combination of the body, the senses, the mind, and the soul. Vedas are ancient Hindu books of knowledge that are said to have been divinely revealed to the sages of India thousands of years ago. There are four Vedas, and ayurveda is related to the fourth, which includes detailed information on the treatment of the sick using mantras, herbs, and potions.

To receive the benefits of ayurveda you don't need to convert to Hinduism or become its advocate. Ayurvedic practitioners only ask that you keep an open mind and have a genuine desire to be healed. Ayurveda is a system of medicine that is gaining popularity and acceptance in the West and can work alongside Western medical practices.

Working under the ancient precept to do no harm, ayurvedic practitioners prescribe remedies derived from natural substances that are highly effective and nontoxic.

The ayurvedic philosophy is based on permanent, timeless, and wise principles of living and encourages a good and moral way of life. Morality promotes harmony, which in turn promotes health and happiness.

A number of ayurvedic principles form the groundwork to maintain harmony and wellness. Based on Hindu teachings, ayurveda submits five rules of conduct that need to be followed. If any of the rules are broken, a disorder, or illness, results.

Five Principles of Conduct

The first rule is to avoid killing. Humans are considered to be the guardians of all living things, and to shed the blood of another creature is wrong. Therefore, ayurvedic medical treatments are generally vegetarian. In cases where a patient requires a certain kind of protein that can't be obtained in any other manner, an ayurvedic practitioner may prescribe meat to be included in the diet.

The second rule is to avoid stealing and lying. Since stealing and lying are inherently considered to be wrong, to do so creates tension and disharmony. Not only do others suffer as a result of the action, but the fear of getting caught affects the health of the perpetrator.

The third rule is to avoid sexual misconduct. The actual definition of "sexual misconduct" carries a different meaning today than it did thousands of years ago, in keeping with social development and what is now considered acceptable. Originally, sex was considered a strictly biological function, and any sexual activity that didn't end with the ultimate goal of procreation was considered misconduct. Today an ayurvedic practitioner would consider a sexual activity that might harm or exploit another person (or oneself) as sexual misconduct. Sexually transmitted and stress-related diseases are generally considered to be a result of promiscuity.

Keep in mind that ayurveda is the first system of medicine to acknowledge the importance of individual sexuality. Although it's also important to remember that in the origins of ayurveda only men were considered to have a sex drive and women were apathetic to sexual activity.

The fourth rule is to avoid alcohol. Once again, during the space of thousands of years, this rule has been modified to reflect current conditions and societal changes.

When the ayurvedic texts were compiled, alcohol was pretty much the only mind-altering chemical, in beverage form,

8 • Gymnema

available. Now, of course, we have the ubiquitous coffee, as well as a wide range of sodas, colas, and other processed sugary drinks that contain the stimulant caffeine. Ayurvedic practitioners consider these drinks to be on par with alcohol. Although in specific cases, such as someone with high cholesterol, moderate intake of alcohol may be suitable.

The fifth rule is the doctrine of the "middle road," or moderation in all things.

Ayurveda's Eight Branches

Ayurveda encompasses eight specialties: internal medicine, pediatrics, *rasayana* or "rejuvenator," toxicology, psychiatry, *vajikarna* or aphrodisiacs, ENT/ophthalmology, and surgery.

If you are studying the art of ayurveda, you may find it difficult to distinguish between rasayana and vajikarna. Since a healthy sexual system is dependent upon a properly functioning mind and body, the two are inextricably linked. The difference lies in the remedies: initially for rasayana, the patient was prescribed herbal dietary supplements, while vajikarna prescriptions were comprised of poisons, narcotics, animal products, and minerals.

For a health-care system that is thousands of years old, ayurveda remains relevant to "modern" ailments such as irritable bowel syndrome, depression, and stress-related illnesses. Although traditional ayurvedic medicine included surgery, modern-day practitioners concede that Western surgical techniques are far more advanced and now focus primarily on improving health through balance.

Balance

Balance is a key principle in ayurveda. A fundamental philosophy of ayurveda is the concept of *tridoshas* or the three bioenergies (*doshas*) that exist in all living matter. Any imbalance in the three doshas results in illness in the body or mind.

A loose equivalent of the tridoshas is the Western catego-

History of Ayurveda • 9

rization of body types: endomorph (stocky) or *kapha*; meso-morph (muscular and compact) or *pitta*; and ectomorph (lean and delicate) or *vata*.

The doshas describe more than just body types, they also describe personality preferences and predispositions. Doshas have both positive and negative qualities. For example, kapha individuals have patient, stable personalities and are slow to anger. They also tend to be slow, almost lethargic, in their actions and speech. A pitta individual is open to new ideas and has a precise and irritable disposition. He or she is also intellectual and articulate. A vata individual is thin and not prone to weight gain, but is nervous and restless.

Rarely do people fall solely into one of the three categories; most people are a combination of the three, and within the combination a dominant dosha usually exists. Rarely do people display the characteristics of their dominant dosha in a pure, undiluted form.

Pitta and kapha are respectively considered the destructive and creative forces of the universe, while vata regulates the interactions between them. Using this basic philosophy, ayurvedic practitioners are able to relate it to the human body regarding many issues, from general to specific.

As stated in the *Susruta Samhita* over two thousand years ago, "Vata, Pitta and Kapha are the primary essential principles animating the human organism. . . . The human body is supported by the three fundamental principles in the same way a house is supported by its foundation."

The various functions of our bodies are attributed to the doshas and the properties they possess.

Our bodies' nervous system, motor activities, and movement are considered *vata*. The symptoms an ayurvedic practitioner would look for with a vata dosha are sharp pain, shooting pulse, dryness, coldness, and nervous movement, among others. Sweet and nourishing herbs are generally used to correct imbalances. The herbs would strengthen the digestive system and be calming and moisturizing. Commonly used are ashwagandha root, bala, and gokshura fruit.

Pitta relates to metabolism, removing metabolic wastes from the system, and the body's chemical processes (enzymes and hormones). Symptoms of a kapha imbalance include excessive heat, burning pain, racing pulse, and strong odors. Pitta herbs are generally cooling, detoxifying, astringent, and nourishing. Commonly used herbs are licorice root, boswellia, turmeric root, and neem leaves.

Kapha includes the circulatory, skeletal, and anabolic systems, and basically the entire physical construction of the body. Disorders almost always result from the body's difficulty in delivering nutrients via the arteries to the tissues and organs that need them. An excess production of mucus is also a kapha disorder. Herbs used to bring about balance are usually astringent, warming, mucus reducing, and cooling. Commonly used are guggul, turmeric root, black pepper, and vidanga seeds.

Ayurveda is based on the central belief that all is One— everything in existence is related and linked and lives in a relative balance and harmony. When this harmony is disrupted in a patient—in physical, spiritual, or psychological manner—illness is a result.

A practitioner will assess a person's physical condition and lifestyle and will determine where and how the imbalance is manifesting itself. By identifying a dosha's effect, the practitioner will then try to counter its harmful influences.

Practitioners attempt to reestablish balance with herbs, diet, lifestyle, yoga, meditation, *marma* puncture (ayurvedic acupuncture), or a combination of any of the above.

Herbal remedies in ayurvedic medicine are administered in pure herbal form, not manufactured or processed in a laboratory. Rarely are single herbs used in a remedy. Combinations of herbs are used to work together in a synergistic fashion. Most ayurvedic medicines contain between five and twenty-five ingredients, mostly herbs and minerals.

Gymnema (*Gymnema sylvestre*)

The gymnema plant is a vine with egg-shaped leaves and yellow flower clusters. Gymnema is indigenous to tropical Asian forests.

The first documented use of gymnema to control hyperglycemia was in the 1920s. Gymnema performs a "sugar blocking" action on both the taste buds and also the small intestine by blocking the paths that sugar molecules would normally take, temporarily blocking the absorption of sugar.

Ayurvedic healers may have been the first to notice and recognize diabetes as a disease. Their word for it is *madhumeha*, or "honey urine" because they noticed that ants were attracted to the urine of patients affected with diabetes. Although they didn't know about insulin production or resistance, they noticed that diabetes typically affected two types of *doshas*, or body and digestive types.

The first type of patient, similar to the type 1 diabetic of today, is *vata*, or nerve-natured. The second type, or type 2 diabetic, is *pitta-kapha* and is obese and has a strong appetite. The physique types, eating habits, and demeanor are typical of patients who would be diagnosed with diabetes today.

When ayurvedic practitioners noticed either one of the types of patients afflicted with madhumeha, they would turn to gymnema, usually in combination with other herbs, to reduce blood in the urine and aid digestion.

Gymnema reduces hyperglycemia (high blood sugar) in a number of ways. It stimulates the regeneration of pancreatic cells that produce insulin, thereby producing more insulin; it stimulates the production of enzymes that help the uptake of glucose into cells; and it prevents the stimulation of the liver to produce more glucose.

Several studies conducted in 1990 found that gymnema worked so well in managing blood glucose levels that some diabetes patients could discontinue their prescription medications.

Another study of the effects of gymnema on blood glucose,

plasma insulin, and carbohydrate metabolic enzymes was conducted on diabetic rats. For three weeks, the rats were given an alcoholic extract of gymnema (called GS4). Tests showed that their body weight and blood glucose levels decreased and their plasma insulin levels increased significantly.

In 2001, during the course of twelve herbal medicine education seminars in Italy, 720 questionnaires were distributed asking herbalists what they would recommend to their patients for different ailments. In the 685 responses received, gymnema led the list of the top-ten recommendations for controlling hyperglycemia (the other nine are mentioned in a later chapter).

The advantage of gymnema over prescription medications for diabetes is that gymnema can control blood glucose levels without bringing them below normal levels, unlike some of the prescription medications.

What Is Diabetes?

Diabetes is a metabolic disorder that affects twenty million Americans. Of those, about one-third have not been diagnosed. Each year, over a million people over twenty are diagnosed with the disease.

When we eat food, our bodies break down the food into glucose, which is our body's fuel. After the food is digested, the glucose that's produced passes into the bloodstream, where it's absorbed by cells to be used for energy and growth. The cells need insulin so they can absorb the glucose.

Insulin is a hormone that's produced by the pancreas. Normally, the pancreas produces enough insulin for the body to absorb glucose. In diabetics, however, the pancreas either doesn't produce enough insulin, or the cells don't properly utilize existing insulin. The excess glucose then builds up in the blood and is passed into the urine where it leaves the body.

When glucose doesn't enter cells properly and builds up in

the blood, two problems can result: Cells are starved for energy. Long-term high blood glucose levels damage the eyes, kidneys, nerves, heart, and feet.

Symptoms of Diabetes

- Thirst
- Frequent urination
- Weight loss
- Increased appetite
- Blurred vision
- Irritability
- Tingling or numbness in the hands or feet
- Frequent skin, bladder, or gum infections
- Wounds that don't heal
- Extreme fatigue

People with type 2 diabetes frequently have no symptoms. Type 2 diabetes progresses so gradually that it might not be noticed by the patient for years.

Diagnosing Diabetes

To diagnose diabetes or pre-diabetes (also closely related to metabolic syndrome or syndrome-X), a fasting plasma glucose test (FPG) or an oral glucose tolerance (OGTT) test is performed.

With the fasting plasma glucose test, a result of 100 and 125 mg/dl indicates pre-diabetes. If the score is 126 mg/dl or higher, the patient has diabetes. With the oral glucose tolerance test, a patient fasts and drinks a glucose/water solution. Two hours later, the blood glucose level is tested. If the patient's results are from 140 to 199 mg/dl, the patient has pre-diabetes. Higher than 200 mg/dl indicates diabetes.

Risk Factors for Diabetes

Heredity: Unfortunately, gymnema cannot compensate for a genetic predisposition to contracting diabetes.

Obesity: In an eight-week study of sixty moderately obese patients, gymnema has shown effectiveness in regulating weight and blood sugar levels. One third of the study's participants were given 400 mg of gymnema three times a day along with a 2,000 calorie per day diet and moderate exercise. By the end of eight weeks, the patients showed a decrease in body weight and body mass index (BMI) of 5–6 percent as well as a significant decrease in total cholesterol, low-density lipoproteins, and serum leptin levels.

High cholesterol

High blood pressure

Physical inactivity

Advancing age

Ethnicity: People of Native American, African American, Hispanic, Asian, and Pacific Island descent.

Types of Diabetes

While we don't currently understand the all the underlying causes of diabetes, genetics and environment seem to play an important role. Diabetes can be divided into four types:

- Type 1
- Type 2
- Gestational diabetes
- Pre-diabetes

Type 1

In type 1 diabetes, the body does not produce insulin. Previously known as juvenile-onset diabetes, type 1 diabetes is usually diagnosed in children and young adults. Patients diagnosed with type 1 diabetes usually require a diet high in protein, vegetables, and healthy fats, with restrictions on sugar and carbohydrates (particularly refined carbohydrates).

Type 2

In type 2 diabetes, the most common form, the body develops a resistance to insulin or doesn't produce adequate amounts of insulin. Some populations are more prone to developing type 2 diabetes, and the number of adolescents who develop type 2 diabetes is growing.

Type 2 diabetes is associated with excess weight and a diet rich in refined carbohydrates (white sugar, high-fructose corn syrup, white flour, etc.) and lacking in healthy fruits and vegetables. The incidence of type 2 diabetes is higher in countries that eat a diet similar to the basic American diet, with lots of simple sugars.

Gestational Diabetes

Gestational diabetes affects 4 percent of pregnant women. The hormones that develop to support the growth of a fetus may block the mother's insulin action, also called insulin resistance. With this kind of resistance, the mother's body may need up to three times the normal amount of insulin. When inadequate quantities of insulin are produced, blood sugar levels increase and lead to gestational diabetes.

Once diagnosed, treatment must begin immediately to protect the lives and health of mother and child. Treatment includes special meal plans and exercise, and the condition may need to be controlled with insulin. A woman who develops gestational diabetes has increased chances of developing type 2 diabetes later in life.

Pre-Diabetes

Pre-diabetes is indicated by high levels of blood glucose, but not high enough to indicate type 2 diabetes. People diagnosed with type 2 diabetes typically had pre-diabetes before their diagnosis. Through the course of pre-diabetes, long-term damage is being inflicted on the cardiovascular and circulatory systems.

Early intervention and treatment of pre-diabetes can prevent the onset of type 2 diabetes. By adhering to a rigorous exercise program and changing the diet by strictly limiting all refined carbohydrates and increasing the intake of fresh fruits and vegetables and healthy low-fat protein sources such as fish and chicken, type 2 diabetes doesn't have to be inevitable. Taking one of the glucose tests mentioned above is the best way to determine if you have pre-diabetes.

Managing Blood Glucose Levels

Managing blood glucose levels effectively is of critical importance in the life of every diabetic. When the body doesn't have enough insulin, it begins to break down fats for fuel. This process stimulates a production of waste called ketones. The body cannot tolerate excessive quantities of ketones and will try to eliminate them in the urine. If the body can't expel enough ketones in the urine, they will build up and lead to a condition called ketoacidosis.

Found primarily in type 1 diabetics, ketoacidosis—otherwise known as diabetic coma—is a life-threatening condition that requires immediate treatment. Ketoacidosis is characterized by dry mouth, nausea and vomiting, shortness of breath, and fruity-smelling breath. If you suspect that you're experiencing ketoacidosis, seek immediate medical attention.

Hypoglycemia

Hypoglycemia, or low blood sugar, can be prevented by adequately controlling blood sugar levels. But if it does occur, hypoglycemia must be treated immediately. How do you know if you're hypoglycemic? Symptoms include: shakiness, dizziness, sweating, hunger, headaches, skin pallor, moodiness and irritability, tingly sensations around the mouth, and poor concentration. The fastest way to treat hypoglycemia is to ingest some form of sugar (such as skim milk or fruit juice), which will increase blood glucose to normal levels. It's critical to learn to recognize the symptoms of hypoglycemia so it can be treated promptly. And it's important to make sure that you always have some type of snack close at hand if hypoglycemia should strike. Untreated hypoglycemia can lead to unconsciousness, which could have life-threatening consequences, particularly while driving.

Hyperglycemia

Hyperglycemia, conversely, is elevated blood sugar levels. This is a serious condition and is most common among people with diabetes. Blood sugar levels may become elevated in type 1 patients if they didn't inject enough insulin, and in type 2 patients if their insulin isn't being properly utilized by the body. Hyperglycemia can also be caused by stress, lack of exercise, overeating, and illness. Symptoms include increased thirst and frequent urination.

Patients with type 2 diabetes sometimes experience a condition called hyperosmolar hyperglycemic nonketotic syndrome, or HHNS. HHNS typically occurs in older people as the result of illness. As blood sugar levels rise, the body tries to eliminate excess sugar by passing it into the urine. Symptoms of HHNS include very high blood sugar levels (600 mg/dl and over), dry mouth, increased thirst, high fever, confusion, loss of vision, and warm, dry skin. If you have any of these symptoms, you should seek medical attention immediately.

Treating Diabetes

The best way to treat diabetes is by strictly controlling blood sugar levels. Regularly checking blood sugar levels and maintaining tight control is the responsibility of each diabetic. To keep blood sugar within safe parameters, proper diet and exercise are essential. If diet and exercise are not sufficient, some diabetics will need to take insulin or other appropriate medications as prescribed by their physicians.

Long-Term Complications

Effectively managing diabetes requires a disciplined, long-term commitment to responsibly and consistently caring for oneself—through diet, exercise, frequent blood sugar testing, and managing stress. If diabetes is not managed properly, serious complications can result, including:

Heart disease

Stroke

Blindness: Cataracts are the leading cause of blindness worldwide, and diabetes is a major risk factor. Tissue disruption is probably caused by the high sugar levels. In animal studies, scientists used an herbal remedy, which included gymnema, to study its cataract-inhibiting effects. The conclusion is that gymnema is very effective in protecting the eye's lens against sugar-induced cataracts.

Kidney failure

Blood vessel disease resulting in amputation, nerve damage, and impotence.

Depression

Foot complications

Skin complications

Caring for Yourself

Quit smoking: Absolutely essential to improve your health and control your diabetes.

Regular daily exercise: Exercise will lower blood sugar levels, improve circulation and metabolism, strengthen your cardio-vascular system, and burn fat. All of these benefits will help you fight off other diabetes-related symptoms.

Proper foot care: Includes an annual foot examination by a podiatrist or other medical professional, a daily foot self-examination, daily washing, and proper nail trimming. Diabetics should *never* go barefoot, even indoors, and should avoid wearing any type of shoes, socks, or stockings that are too tight. See your podiatrist or physician for complete foot-care instructions.

Relaxation and stress reduction: Lower stress levels can lead to lower blood sugar levels and a decreased need for medication. Ways to reduce stress include meditation, t'ai chi, conscious breathing, biofeedback, deep muscle relaxation, therapeutic massage, and adequate amounts of sleep.

Eye care: Since diabetics are more prone to retinopathy, glaucoma, and cataracts, an annual eye exam by a good ophthalmologist is critical. Strictly managing blood sugar levels and consistent self-care will help forestall or prevent diabetes-related eye problems.

To control type 1 diabetes, some practitioners say that gymnema is preferable to, or can be an adjunct to, injectable insulin. Consult with your diabetes specialist to determine if gymnema might be an effective part of your diabetes treatment program.

Gymnema and Other Conditions

Gymnema is used by ayurvedic practitioners to treat other ailments, including malaria, constipation, digestive problems, and coughs. Preliminary animal studies also indicate that gymnema may be effective in lowering levels of "bad" or LDL cholesterol.

As a folk remedy, gymnema has been used to treat stomachaches, anemia, hyperactivity, urinary tract infections, eye inflammation, fever, obesity, scaly skin, and snakebite.

Gymnema Dosage

Gymnema can take several weeks to have therapeutic effects, so continue taking it until the desired response is achieved. Gymnema is available in many forms: dried, powdered, or fresh leaves, capsules, tablets, and liquid extract. In capsule form, the recommended dosage is 400 mg three times a day with meals.

Precautions

While gymnema is considered to be very safe, consult with your physician before including it as part of your health-care regimen. Gymnema may increase insulin levels in healthy, non-diabetic people and may decrease iron absorption. It's essential that people diagnosed with type 1 or type 2 diabetes discuss gymnema with their physician before adding it to their treatment plan.

Herbs Commonly Used to Control Blood Sugar Levels

Psyllium (*Plantago psyllium*): One of the safest, gentlest laxatives available. Psyllium is the active ingredient in the name-brand product Metamucil. Recent research suggests that psyllium may help reduce cholesterol levels. It can be used to treat diarrhea, constipation, hemorrhoids, and high cholesterol. Psyllium's high fiber content may help reduce the risk of colon cancer. Take a teaspoon or two of psyllium three times a day, with at least 12 ounces of water or juice. Do not give to children under age two.

Fenugreek (*Foenum-graecum*): Historically, fenugreek has played a major healing role and was even found in the tomb of King Tut. It's used to decrease cholesterol levels, lower blood sugar levels, relieve sore throats, treat wounds, treat arthritis, and help with women's health issues. Fenugreek seeds contain diosgenin, which is similar to estrogen, suggesting that it could be used as a natural form of hormone replacement therapy. It may be a uterine stimulant, so pregnant women should not take it.

Bilberry (*Vaccinium myrtillus*): Sometimes called European blueberries, bilberry has been used in herbal healing for over eight hundred years. During World War II, British aviators discovered bilberry's true treasure: preventing night blindness and sharpening night vision. Bilberries are powerful antioxidants and help prevent cell damage caused by free radicals. Bilberries can be used for general disease prevention, and can prevent and inhibit cataracts, improve macular degeneration, improve diabetic retinopathy, and treat varicose veins. Some studies suggest that bilberries help lower blood sugar levels.

Garlic (*Allium sativum*): In the world of natural healing, garlic is considered to be a wonder drug. It's a very powerful healing agent and is used to cure a host of ills. Garlic is used to fight infections, treat ulcers, lower cholesterol, and is considered to have anticarcinogenic properties. As a disease-prevention agent, garlic is used to prevent arterial hardening, high cholesterol, and high blood pressure. It's also been shown to lower blood sugar and can be used in the treatment of diabetes.

Chinese ginseng (*Panax quinquefolium*): Chinese ginseng had been the subject of over 1,500 books, and it has been used for its medicinal and adaptogenic properties for centuries. In a study of thirty-six newly diagnosed type 2 diabetics, participants who were given ginseng reported a greater improvement in mood, increased performance on physical and psychological tests, and lower blood sugar levels than the control group. Chinese ginseng has also been used to improve well-being, increase energy, enhance athletic performance, enhance immunity, and improve mental acuity.

Dandelion (*Taraxacum officinale*): More than a weed to healers, dandelion has been used as a treatment for over a thousand years. It reportedly can prevent gallstones, ease the symptoms of pre-menstrual syndrome, reduce blood pressure, prevent cell damage that leads to cancer, inhibit yeast infections, and eliminate water weight. Recent studies have shown that it may help reduce blood sugar levels.

Burdock (*Arctium lappa*): Early Chinese physicians and ayurvedic practitioners used burdock to treat colds, throat infections, flu, and pneumonia. Recent studies show that it may have antitumor properties. Although not backed by scientific research, herbalists believe that burdock is a blood purifier and can lower blood sugar levels.

Prickly pear cactus (*Opuntia humifusa*): This herbal remedy is taken from the fruits and pads of the succulent plant that grows in desert regions. Prickly pear is rich in slowly absorbed soluble fibers that may help stabilize blood sugar levels.

Bitter melon (*Momordica charantia*): Scientific studies in the early stages are looking at bitter melon as a treatment for diabetes, cancer, and HIV.

Other Herbs Used to Control Blood Sugar Levels

Aloe (*Aloe vera*): Commonly used to treat minor burns and cuts, aloe juice has shown to lower glucose levels in humans and animals.

Apple (*Pyrus malus*): "An apple a day . . ." Pectin in apples has been proven to help reduce blood sugar, in addition to providing fiber to the recommended high-fiber diet.

Blackberry (*Rubus fructicosus*): The substance that gives blackberries their rich color also contains powerful antioxidants. Blackberries assist in cell regeneration and protection and improve the damage cased by diabetic retinopathy. One study also found that a strong tea made from blackberry leaves reduced blood sugar levels.

Black cohosh (*Cimicifuga racemosa*): known as the "women's herb," black cohosh has been used to treat pre-menstrual syndrome, menstrual cramps, and menopause. Other research indicates that it may be used to lower cholesterol, blood pressure, and blood sugar levels, all of which are very important in managing diabetes.

Celery (*Apium graveolens*): The stalks and seeds of celery can be used to treat gout, high blood pressure, high cholesterol, congestive heart failure, and diabetes. Celery seeds have been used to reduce blood sugar levels.

Cinnamon (*Cinnamomum zeylanicum*): Found in ancient Chinese texts on herbal medicines dating back about four thousand years, cinnamon has been used for a variety of purposes including medicinal, culinary, and practical. As one of the oldest remedies in traditional Chinese medicine, cinnamon has been used to treat a variety of ailments, including diarrhea, influenza, and parasitic worms.

Cinnamon is a potent antifungal and antibacterial agent. It helps with type 2 diabetes by moderating blood sugar levels. Cinnamon also lowers cholesterol, and its very smell is considered a brain booster! Be sure to use true cinnamon (*Cinnamomum zeylanicum*), not cassia, which is typically labeled as cinnamon.

Ginger (*Zingiber officinale*): Ginger is used by pregnant women to reduce the nausea and vomiting associated with morning sickness. It's antinausea properties make it ideal for treating vertigo, dizziness, and motion sickness. Fresh ginger is more effective against nausea than powdered ginger, but powdered ginger is more effective in warming the body.

Ginger has active ingredients that may act as an analgesic and anti-inflammatory. Ginger lowers the body's level of natural pain-causing compounds called prostaglandins. It can be taken either in standardized capsule form, as a powder, or as a topical massage oil. As a warming agent, ginger is also used to increase poor circulation.

Juniper (*Juniperus communis*): Juniper is being used to treat high blood pressure, congestive heart failure, and arthritis. Initial animal studies show that juniper reduces blood sugar levels.

Other Herbs Used to Control Blood Sugar Levels • 25

Marshmallow (*Althaea officinalis*): Used as a treatment for wounds, respiratory problems, and for enhancing immunity, marshmallow has been shown in recent studies to be useful in managing diabetes because of its ability to lower blood sugar levels.

Raspberry (*Rubus idaeus*): Raspberries are a powerful antioxidant. Raspberry leaf tea is a traditional remedy for diarrhea. One animal study so far has indicated that it helps lower blood sugar levels.

Sage (*Salvia officinalis*): Sage has been around for thousands of years and is used as a remedy for many maladies, including wounds, food poisoning, digestive problems, and sore throats. A German study found that diabetic patients who were able to drink sage tea on an empty stomach were able to lower their blood sugar levels.

Turmeric (*Curcuma longa*): A member of the ginger family, turmeric has been shown to have anti-inflammatory properties. Turmeric is a strong antioxidant that boosts immunity and can be used as part of an herbal regimen for overall wellness. As a folk remedy, turmeric has been used to treat wounds and scabies, to fight salmonella, prevent cataracts, prevent cell damage caused by cancer, and fight heart disease and liver damage. Turmeric may lower blood sugar levels and prevent ulcers and gallstones.

References

American Diabetes Association Web site: www.diabetes.org.

Ananthan, R., M. Latha, L. Pari, K. M. Ramkumar, C. G. Baskar, V. N. Bai. "Effect of *Gymnema montanum* on blood glucose, plasma insulin, and carbohydrate metabolic enzymes in alloxan-induced diabetic rats." *J-Med-Food*, 2003 Spring; 6 (1): 43–49.

Bratman, Steven, M.D., and Andrea M. Girman, M.D., M.P.H. *Mosby's Handbook of Herbs and Supplements and their Therapeutic Uses*, 2003.

Castleman, Michael. *The New Healing Herbs: The Classic Guide to Nature's Best Medicines*, 2001.

Chopra, Deepak. *Ageless Body, Timeless Mind*,1993.

Cicero, A. F., G. Derosa, A. Gaddi. "What do herbalists suggest to diabetic patients in order to improve glycemic control? Evaluation of scientific evidence and potential risks." *Acta-Diabetol*, 2004 Sep; 41 (3): 91–98.

Duke, James A., Ph.D. *The Green Pharmacy Herbal Handbook*, 2000.

Fields, Gregory P. *Religious Therapeutics: Body and Health in Yoga, Ayurveda, and Tantra*, 2001.

Godagama, Shantha. *The Handbook of Ayurveda*, 1997.

IBIDS Database, National Institutes of Health, Office of Dietary Supplements, Jan. 2006.

Mandile, Maria Noel. *Natural Health*, July 2003, vol. 33, p. 65 (9).

Moghaddam, M. S., P. A. Kumar, G. B. Reddy, V. S. Ghole, *J-Ethnopharmacol*, 2005 Feb. 29: 97 (2): 397–403.

Natural Medicines Comprehensive Database, Fourth Edition, 2002.

Pedersen, Mark. *Nutritional Herbology: A Reference Guide to Herbs*, 1995.

Preuss, J. G., D. Bagchi, M. Bagchi, C. V. Rao, D. K. Dey, S. Satyanarayana. "Effects of a natural extract of (-) hydroxycitric acid and a combination of HCA-SX plus niacin-bound chromium and *Gymnema sylvestre* extract on weight *loss*." *Diabetes-Obes-Metab*. 2004 May; 6 (3): 171–180.

Puri, Harbans Singh. *Rasayana: Ayurvedic Herbs for Longevity and Rejuvenation: Traditional Herbal Medicines for Modern Times*, Vol. 2, 2003.

Ritchason, Jack, N.D. *The Little Herb Encyclopedia*, Third Edition, 1995.

Tillotsen, Alan Keith, Ph.D. *The One Earth Herbal Sourcebook: Everything You Need To Know About Chinese, Western, and Ayurvedic Herbal Treatments*, 2001